Praise for Timothy A. Carey's
HOLD THAT THOUGHT!

"Tim Carey was the first person to train, supervise, and evaluate Method of Levels therapy in everyday clinical practice. The implications of the technique for psychotherapy integration, service organization, and service-user recovery and empowerment are staggering. Dr. Carey has now managed another first – an engaging, accessible therapy manual that is scientifically grounded and pioneering, all within 141 pages!"

Dr. Warren Mansell
Senior Lecturer in Psychology, Clinical Psychologist,
and Cognitive Behavioral Therapist
University of Manchester
Manchester, United Kingdom

"This book is an immediately useable, practical guide for anyone in a helping practice, no matter what their previous training. It is a fascinating process that will blow you away with its simplicity and yet stun you with the profound depth it can reach."

Jenny McFadden
Counselor, Lecturer, and Instructor for
Association for Applied Control Theory Australia

"This form of therapy is exciting – first because of its simplicity and speed, and second because the therapist gets to observe a moment of transformation as the client perceives the conflict at a different level."

Judy McFadden
Psychologist, Author, Senior Faculty Member of
Association for Applied Control Theory Australia

OTHER TITLES BY TIMOTHY A. CAREY

The Method of Levels: How to do Psychotherapy Without Getting in the Way

RTP Intervention Processes,
with Margaret Carey

COMING SOON FROM TIMOTHY A. CAREY

Something for Teachers
(Who Want to be Revolutionaries)

Hold That Thought!

HOLD THAT THOUGHT!

Two Steps to Effective Counseling and
Psychotherapy with the Method of Levels

Timothy A. Carey

newview
St. Louis, MO

Hold That Thought: Two Steps to Effective Counseling and Psychotherapy with the Method of Levels. Copyright ©2008 by Timothy A. Carey. All rights reserved. Printed in the United States of America. No part of this book may be used or reproduced in any manner whatsoever without written permission except in the case of brief quotations embodied in critical articles or reviews. For information, address newview, 10 Dover Lane, Villa Ridge, Missouri 63089-2001, (800) 441-3604.

Cover photograph by Patrick Carey.

Cover design and interior layout by Scott Byerly.

Illustrations by Josh Taylor.

ISBN 0-944337-49-X.

For Jack

I hope by the time you're old enough to understand these words a whole lot of the rest of the world does too.

Thanks

I am grateful to the friends and colleagues who have helped me put this book together. Tom Bourbon, Bill Powers, Rick Marken, Phil Runkel, and Dag Forssell have each contributed to my knowledge of PCT in different and important ways. Bill also provided coaching and mentoring while I was learning MOL.

Richard and Gillian Mullan and Chris and Margaret Spratt, as revolutionary pioneers, jumped aboard and demonstrated that MOL wasn't an idiosyncrasy of one therapist but could be learned and used successfully by others. Sara Tai's interest and involvement has been enormously encouraging also. It was a throw away comment by Gillian one night at a fun-filled preconference dinner in Manchester that led to the title of this book.

Warren Mansell has been instrumental in the United Kingdom in opening doors for PCT and

MOL in both applied and academic settings.

I was fortunate that David Aaron, Ally Gunn, Peter Marcon, Judy McFadden, Jenny McFadden, June Myatt, Kate Rimes, Shelley Roy, and Thea Vanags took the time to read this manuscript and suggest how it could be improved.

Fred Good was responsible for initially proposing the idea of a book like this and he and his publishing partner Lloyd Klinedinst have done a great job in producing what you're now holding.

I am grateful to have been able to use the amazing cartoon wizardry of Josh Taylor. His efforts have added another wonderfully enjoyable dimension to this book. So too did Scott Byerly's. His stunning sense of design and eye for detail transformed a Word document into the publication you're now holding.

My brother, Patrick, took a superb photo on an isolated beach near St. Andrews in Scotland. That photo is the cover of this book.

Margaret is a PCT student, MOL therapist, proofreader, critic, and friend. By an enormous stroke of good fortune she's also my wife. Thanks for being here and being you.

Contents

Foreword: A Theory and a Method xvii

Why the Method of Levels? xxi

How This Book Works................... xxv

CHAPTER ONE
Business as Usual......................... 1

CHAPTER TWO
A Closer Look at Control 11

CHAPTER THREE
Trouble at the Office.....................21

CHAPTER FOUR
It's Multistory Trouble....................31

CHAPTER FIVE
An Untangling Tool 41

CHAPTER SIX
Finding the Right Place for the Tool 51

CHAPTER SEVEN
Helping MOL Style 61

CHAPTER EIGHT
More About Helping....................71

CHAPTER NINE
Ready, Steady, Up 81

CHAPTER TEN
Right Here, Right Now 93

CHAPTER ELEVEN
Even Not Having a Topic is a Topic........103

CHAPTER TWELVE
In the Absence of Disruptions 115

CHAPTER THIRTEEN
A Special Kind of Helping 125

CHAPTER FOURTEEN
Over to You...........................135

Check these out if you
want to know more 143

Foreword

A Theory and a Method
William T. Powers

This is a book for practical people, not theoreticians. Yet as a theoretician, I can say that it is one of the best expositions of Perceptual Control Theory that you are likely to find. When Dr. Timothy Carey asked me to write a foreword, I read the manuscript and immediately had a problem. The problem is that if you push on a control system, it will push back, even if you're aiding its efforts (if you help too much it relaxes or perversely reverses its efforts). So if I were to reveal my full enthusiasm for this remarkable tutorial on PCT and the Method of Levels, the most likely result in the reader would be just the opposite of what I want. I will therefore refrain from gushing and hyperbole, and merely say that there is no sentence in this book that is there accidentally, or that can be skipped without losing something. It will reward a second reading, and a third. And when you finish it, you will be well on the way to understanding this method, to the point where you can consider trying it with a friend yourself, in either role.

Carey's first handbook on MOL bore the subtitle *How to do Psychotherapy Without Getting in the Way*. That is the theme you will encounter over and over in these pages. Not getting in the way means not doing all those things dear to the fictional therapist in books and on television: having insights into your patient's problem, figuring out what is wrong, and telling your patient what to do about it. If you are getting some practice with being an MOL therapist and fall into those ways, you will see an immediate cessation of progress. Your brilliance will have halted the hard work being done by your client, and turned the spotlight on you, moving your client off the stage into the role of spectator.

In MOL, the therapist is the spectator. The client is the one in the lead, with the therapist acting as a guide who knows where the fish are likely to be, but who has no fishing pole. The guide asks,

"Is that one?" and the client, the explorer in the lead, looks more closely and says, "No, but here's something interesting." Then, with the guide asking helpful but not too suggestive questions, the explorer reels in whatever is on the line for a closer look, letting the guide know what is going on, but not, thank you, requiring any help with the actual landing of the fish. In the Method of Levels, the outcome is the doing of the client, not the therapist.

As a result, the client no longer needs help when similar problems threaten to arise. That is because the client found out how to resolve problems by resolving them, not by following someone else's suggestions. That is a skill that we are all born with, but when a person seeks help, it is because this skill has seemingly stopped working. In MOL sessions, the reason is usually found to be that the wrong thing is being attended to — some effect of the problem rather than its cause. This is what the MOL therapist is good at: helping the client redirect attention toward the cause so the reorganizations accomplish something more than stirring up the mud and obscuring vision. Redirecting attention is something a client can get used to doing even without outside help. That is, or should be, the point of therapy.

Don't be deceived by Timothy Carey's easy language and humor. He is not striving for effect; that is how he is all of the time. That is what makes it possible for him to teach so well, and is also what he has learned by adopting what he calls the 'MOL attitude.' I taught him about the Method of Levels, as a mostly theoretical concept, starting in the mid 1990s. Now he is teaching me, by showing what it is like for a professional therapist to apply the principles all of the time, every day, to everyone, all the while trying to let the process happen and avoid the errors that — temporarily — derail it. You will find all that discussed in the pages to follow, so it is time for me to stop getting in the way.

Bill Powers
April 1, 2008

Why the Method of Levels?

The Method of Levels (MOL) is an application of the principles of Perceptual Control Theory (PCT). PCT has been around since the middle of the twentieth century when William T. Powers (Bill) first started formulating it. PCT is a precise and accurate explanation of how a living thing manages to control those aspects of its life that are necessary or important or both.

With hundreds of psychological therapies available today, however, the introduction of yet another technique could well be met with rolled eyes and impatient sighs. The fact that there *are* so many therapies around is especially relevant to MOL. Given that a good deal of these therapies have been demonstrated to be effective, can it really be the case that they are all so different after all?

Most therapies have their own explanation for how a person becomes troubled and what needs to occur for the trouble to subside. It could happen, therefore, that two people with depression (for example) could access two different therapies with different explanations about their depression and the treatment for it. If both these people resolve their depression, is it likely to be the case that they both had different kinds of depression and, by some extraordinarily fortunate coincidence, each person just happened to turn up to the therapist offering the therapy that matched their particular type of depression? What are the odds of that? Normally, you wouldn't expect depressed people to be that lucky!

A far simpler, and much more probable, explanation is that both people had troubles of a similar nature (although perhaps the specifics were different) and they were able to take what they needed from therapy *despite* the different techniques that were used. My suggestion is that both people took the same thing even though they were given different therapies.

If that sounds a little far fetched, consider for a moment that only a small percentage of all those people who experience troubles that we might call things like depression or social phobia or panic disorder or stress ever get to see a therapist. Most people somehow manage to resolve things without plunging into therapy. Some people might find a book, others might join a club, some might change jobs.

Again, I'm going to suggest that the same thing occurs inside the heads of all those people who move from being psychologically distressed to contented or satisfied *regardless* of the particular way in which they bring about this movement.

It is this internal reordering that MOL targets directly. It can do that because PCT provides a clear and succinct account of what the process is and how it might happen.

The general idea, then, is that rather than MOL being the new kid on the block, it is really the distillation of the effective bit from all those successful therapies. The things that make each therapy distinct belong to the therapies. There is a common essence, however, that is now being utilized directly and explicitly. The utilization is MOL.

So, if you're sure of what you're doing as a therapist and are as about as effective as you want to be, this book won't have much to offer. If, on the other hand, you'd like to be more certain about what this business of helping entails and how you can improve the help you provide, you might find something in these pages of interest.

Welcome!

How This Book Works

There are a number of components to each chapter in this book and I thought it might be useful to explain each one to you.

Underneath the title for each chapter is a question which gives a hint of what you can expect to find out about in that chapter.

Throughout the chapters are little boxes with text. I've used these boxes to add extra information, or provide another example, or explain something in a different way, or clarify a point I've made. They're not essential to the story I'm telling, but they might help make things clearer.

At the end of each chapter I've included a couple of summary points to remind you about what was covered and also to serve as a quick reference when you revisit the book. After the summary points, I've described an activity you could do to help illustrate the material in the chapter.

The important part of each chapter is still the text between the title and the summary. My intention in adding the supporting material is to assist you in digesting the information in each chapter. If you'd still like to know more after reading the chapters and the additional points, there are some web sites and references at the end of the book.

And, after all that, if you still have queries, you'll be like many others of us who have found PCT to be just as important for the questions it provokes as the answers it provides.

Chapter One

Business as Usual

It's just another day at the office

What's life all about?

Have you ever wondered how a creature gets from A to B? It's marvelous isn't it? Puffins fly hundreds of miles from their feeding grounds somewhere in the ocean back to their burrows to lay their eggs. Office workers commute from their homes to their offices. Cheetahs move from their place in the shade to the back of a straggling gazelle.

Arriving at B from A happens

> When I speak about A and B, I'm using them in a very general sense. For example, they might refer to places like your home (A) and the movies (B) or they might refer to points in time like now (A) and a now that hasn't happened yet (B).

over and over during the course of a creature's life, yet how the journey is accomplished is never the same twice. The actions an office worker uses to see himself from his front door to his desk are different everyday. The weather conditions are different, the other people are different, the cars on the road are different. Circumstances almost never repeat, but a creature's intended results do.

Results repeat in all sorts of ways. In fact, our lives are very much the way they are because we are so good at making things happen the way we want rather than the way environmental circumstances would otherwise have them be. I'm not talking about magic

> Sometimes it can seem like factors from the environment make us act in certain ways or put us in particular frames of mind. It's not uncommon to hear expressions like "He brings out the worst in me" or "That always puts a smile on my face." Environmental occurrences, however, are always measured against our own internal sense of "the way we want" and it is this measuring against our personal standards and values — not the occurrence itself — that determines the meaning of the environmental event and, therefore, what comes next. One person's trash is another person's treasure ... that kind of sums it up.

here. Of course we can't make the national lottery results turn out the way we want and we can't spin straw into gold. I'm talking about something much more mundane than vast riches or the fountain of youth.

The "making things happen the way we want" I'm thinking about are the minute to minute, day to day, year to year, birth to death activities of putting our left feet in front of our right and breathing in after we breathe out. Life, in fact, is a constant process of making things happen the way we want. If we take our eye off the ball for very long, sometimes even for just a minute, things will start to change according to the whims of the environment (including other people) and there'll be much work to do once we start paying attention again.

> You can get a sense of how constantly we keep things happening by imagining what might occur if you closed your eyes tightly and counted to ten while you were driving along. What might the state of affairs be once you got to ten and looked out at the world again?

Think how you would look in a week's time if you did nothing between now and then to affect your appearance. No brushing or flossing of teeth, no shaving of faces, no waxing of legs, no tizzying of hair, no showering or bathing, no nothing. This little thought experiment might give you an idea of the constant, invisible (and sometimes not so invisible) forces that we spend our lives counteracting.

For as long as we're warm and breathing we will spend our time making the things we care about happen according to our own desires and wishes rather than according to other forces. This activity of making or keeping things right in the face of environmental jostling is called *control*. This book is about control. People are content or satisfied when they are able to control the things that matter to them. And for most of us, for most of our lives, it's business as usual as far as control is concerned. We wander through our daily happenings pretty much the way we want. Distress and despair appear when control is interfered with or prevented. This book describes one way that people can help others regain control when it has been lost.

Before I discuss the helping that can be done I'd like to linger for a moment on this idea of control. Then I'll outline the problems that can occur and after that I'll talk about how to help someone who has one of these problems and wants some help with it.

Thoughts to Hold

- [ ] From entering to exiting, life involves creating the outcomes we want in constantly and unpredictably changing conditions.

- [ ] Control is the process of using different means to continue experiencing the same end.

Your Turn (if you want one)

Getting a sense of varying our actions to achieve a constant outcome can be easily accomplished. Stand up and lift one foot off the ground. Stand like that for a few moments. Now ... what do you notice?

When I do this I notice that I can easily achieve this stance (the outcome) but while I'm achieving it I can feel lots of goings-on around my ankle, shin, and the sole of my foot (the actions). It doesn't even feel like I'm 'doing' those twitchings. It feels like what I'm doing is standing on one leg.

So, variable actions producing a constant outcome – yep, that's control all right.

Chapter Two

A Closer Look at Control

How does control occur?

Making things happen the way we want is so commonplace that it's easy to miss. Think of the number of vehicles that are on the roads each day. All of those drivers are controlling the speed and position of their cars. Although accidents do happen on the roads these are such a teensy proportion of the total number of trips being made that ac-

> If the ideas in this book are intriguing to you, you can find more details in THE METHOD OF LEVELS: HOW TO DO PSYCHOTHERAPY WITHOUT GETTING IN THE WAY. The idea of control by living things has a growing science behind it based on a theory called Perceptual Control Theory (PCT). PCT was developed by William T. Powers and you can start learning more about the theory with his two books: BEHAVIOR: THE CONTROL OF PERCEPTION and MAKING SENSE OF BEHAVIOR.

cidents are clearly something out of the ordinary (maybe that's why they're called accidents).

Control is so essential to living that it's worth getting to know it better. How *does* a creature get from A to B time and again even though the conditions between A and B are different every time?

In order to arrive at B from anywhere else you have to know that you're not at B. If you think you're already at B, then there'll be no more to do from your perspective even though other people might try and convince you that you're not there yet. People's Bs only ever exist inside their own heads. But knowing you're not at B is not enough. You have to be able to do things to get closer to B. Generally, anything will do as long as it decreases the gap between you and B.

> When I say that Bs exist inside our heads I don't mean that you should sit yourself down in a porch swing and imagine your life away. If I want to visit the Eiffel Tower in Paris I assume there is a Paris with an Eiffel Tower in it that exists independently of my thoughts about it. I'll then set about locating them and positioning myself there. So while we can agree that there is an Eiffel Tower out there somewhere, the wanting to see myself beside it exists only on the inside of me.

And that's about it. Life is a constant process

A Closer Look at Control

of comparing how things are right at this instant with how we want things to be. How does what I'm experiencing compare with what I expect? If they match I'll keep doing what I'm doing. If they don't match I'll do something different.

Little babies control. Babies don't have much going for them in the way of advanced thinking or complicated behavioral repertoires but they know what they want and they know when they're not getting it. They know when they're too wet or too cold or too hungry, and they do whatever they can do – which isn't very much at that age – to make things right.

The cheetah with the gazelle in its sights can't

> Entities that are organized to control by acting to match 'what is' with 'what is wanted' are called control systems. Household heating thermostats and cruise control systems in cars are control systems. In this way, they behave similarly to living things by producing activity (heat or speed) to keep 'what is' (the current temperature or speed) with 'what is wanted' (the temperature or speed setting). An important difference between these control systems and living control systems is that the settings of these control systems are adjusted from outside of them (they never get to say what temperature or speed THEY want) whereas the settings of living control systems can only be adjusted internally.

possibly plan what its actions will be. It has to be able to act in any way it needs to so that the distance between it and the gazelle eventually reaches zero. Control really is about life and death. It's that important.

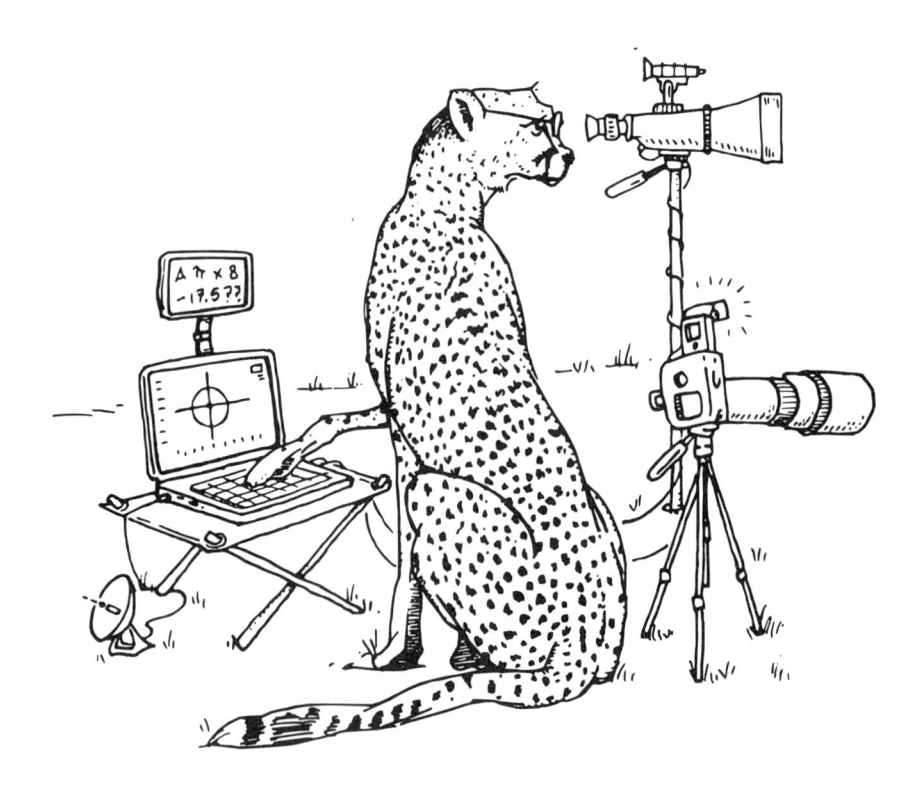

Life then, is like a constant game of 'hotter colder.' Whenever things start to move away from how we'd like them to be we act in whatever way we need to bring them back. W. Thomas Bourbon uses Goldilocks to explain what's going on. At every point in time we know whether things are too hot, too cold, or just right; too hard, too soft, or just right; and so on. Life is the business of making things be just right. We do this by constantly, and often unknowingly, comparing what we're experiencing with what we expect to experience and acting to bring these things to a match and keep them there. At least, that's the normal state of affairs. Sometimes, however, problems occur.

> In this book we'll only be dealing with the 'just rights' that currently exist inside. We won't deal with where 'just rights' come from although you can probably bet it has a lot to do with the qualities we're born with as well as the environments we're born into. If you want to chase that idea further the sources at the end of the book will provide good starting points.

Thoughts to Hold

- Control is the defining characteristic for entities that live.

- Control involves comparing where you are right now with where you want to be and acting in order to make 'right now' the same as 'want to be.'

Your Turn (if you want one)

Have you ever been in the passenger seat of a car with a driver whose 'just right' for the distance between your car and the one in front was different from yours? Was the driver's 'just right' closer to the car in front or further away than yours?

Play around with this ... Have a guess at one of the 'just rights' of someone else and gently 'poke' it. When your friend tells you she likes her coffee with milk and one sugar, serve it to her (as though nothing strange were going on) without milk or sugar. What happens?

Chapter Three

Trouble at the Office

How do problems arise for those who control? (That's all of us!)

Sometimes creatures don't go from A to B. The straggling gazelle didn't get from its grazing place on the savannah to a safe haven. A strong wind might blow a puffin off course or unseen ice on the road might interfere with the car's direction. Occasionally, environmental forces are too great to overcome. You can't roller skate in a buffalo herd – that kind of thing.

> Bush fires, hurricanes, and avalanches are other examples of environmental forces that thwart people's attempts to control.

At other times you might not know where B is. You're in a new town without a map and you have only a few minutes left before the wedding. You bought the latest state-of-the-art gadget but the installation and assembly instructions weren't supplied. Your new boss has taken you out to a ritzy restaurant and there's more cutlery in front of you than you've ever seen before. Where do you start? Sometimes there is no map of the territory.

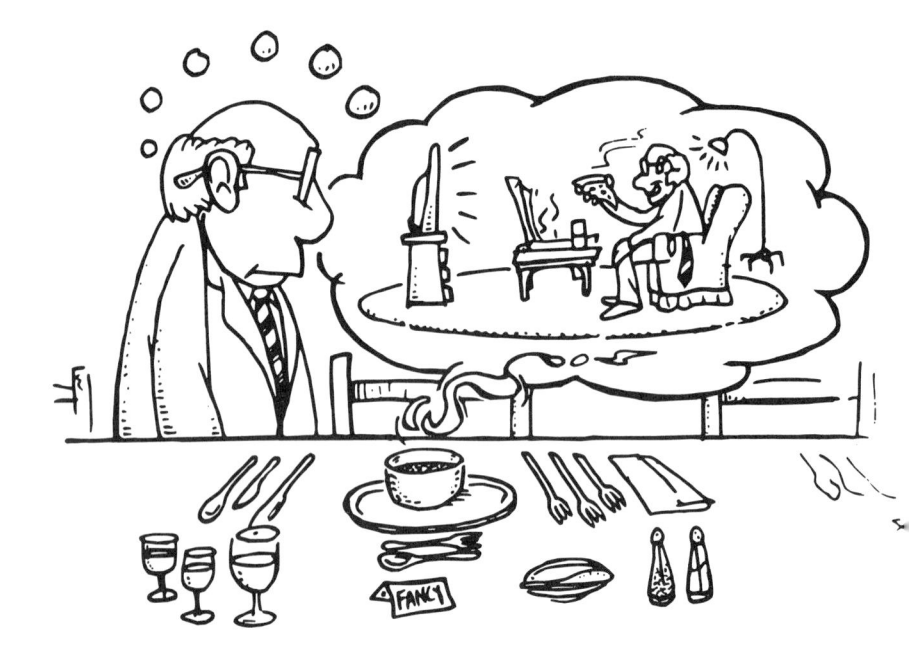

A third situation occurs when there are two Bs in mind. If the two Bs are equally important then the mind will get stuck in the middle of them unable to make either one occur satisfactorily. For the time that this dilemma is in place we can't get either B. Will I have a coffee or put the dinner on?

Will I answer the phone or get the door? Will I order the curry or the stir-fry? Have you ever been stuck in front of the wardrobe holding one shirt in each hand and unable to decide? Do you ever notice yourself dithering between two alternatives?

Each of these situations – overpowering environmental forces, no internal map of the territory, and opposing Bs – can be extremely irksome. The resilience of controlling creatures, however, is astounding. Assuming they actually survive – unlike our lethargic gazelle – things that control eventually find a way to get back on track.

From time to time, however, problems persist. People get stuck and can't get unstuck. When impediments to control endure they are almost always in the form of the third situation. That is, there are two Bs that the person is trying to achieve simultaneously. Will I make my own career decision or do what my parents want? Should I move interstate to be with my new partner or stay with my friends and family? Do I settle for the relationship I've got or start again on my own?

Have you ever had the experience of arguing or fighting with yourself? Any time there is a sense of internal struggling or pushing or resisting there's likely to be conflict going on. Sometimes it feels like a tug-of-war or an arm wrestle inside your head. Sometimes it feels like trying hard to make yourself do one thing rather than something else. Sometimes it's like having two voices in your head – one telling you one thing and the other telling you the opposite. Experiences of conflict vary but the sense of opposition or resistance is common.

> Some of our common expressions convey the notion of two opposing states. "Stuck between a rock and a hard place," "caught between the devil and the deep blue sea," "damned if you do and damned if you don't," and wanting to "have your cake and eat it too" all capture the idea of being pulled or drawn in two opposite directions.

Although not all conflicts persist (*Curry or stir-fry? Hmm, I'll have the curry*), persistent problems are almost always conflicts. Whenever a creature that controls does not get back on track and resume controlling – assuming it's physically able to – odds are that there is a conflict lurking.

So, when people move from a state of distress to greater contentment it is most likely that a conflict has been dissolved. The idea in this book is that helping people extinguish significant psychological distress involves helping them reorganize conflicts. From two Bs to not two Bs – that is the suggestion.

> Throughout this book, when I refer to conflict I am referring to internal conflict. PCT can also help make sense of interpersonal conflict, but conflict BETWEEN people is not the subject of this book. The only conflict I discuss here is conflict WITHIN a person.

Thoughts to Hold

- Problems of control can occur through overwhelming physical forces, the lack of an internal reference, or conflict.

- When problems endure, the nature of the trouble is almost always conflict.

Your Turn (if you want one)

How many times a day do you make choices between two or more alternatives? Keep track of all your choices for a day. Choices are essentially a conflict arrangement — two options but only one will do. How do you make the choice? Is it always the same way?

Do you have a habit you've been trying to change for a long time? Maybe you want to stop smoking, or lose weight, or grow your nails, or exercise more. Have you ever found yourself thinking or saying "I'd love to (lose weight, stop smoking, etc.) but …" What's the but?

Try it the other way around. Say out loud "The thing I absolutely love about (smoking, being the weight I am, etc.) is …" and then notice what comes into your mind.

Chapter Four

It's Multistory Trouble

How are conflicts designed?

The construction of conflicts becomes important when providing an explanation for how to help people remove them. The PCT angle is that conflicts occur across different levels of our experiences. It's not hard to appreciate that some things we experience, like the warmth of the sun, are less complex than other things we experience, like the warmth of another's love.

Getting a sense of this increasing and decreasing complexity is possible through 'why' and 'how' questions. If you think of the answer to "Why are you reading this book?" and then ask "Why?" to whatever the answer to that question is, and then "Why?" to that answer, and then "Why?" again, you might notice that where you're at now is more

> Have you ever been told that 'why' questions should be avoided when counseling? This is where a robust theory comes in handy. 'Why' questions from the perspective of demanding an explanation are not very helpful but, because of the way the hierarchy of levels works according to PCT, 'why' questions can be asked from the point of view of helping people become aware of their higher level goals or purposes.

abstract, more complex, and perhaps even more fundamental than where you started from.

On the other hand, if you ask, "How am I going to read this book?" and then "How?" to the answer of that question, and then "How?" to that answer and so on, you might notice that you've got a lot more specific, perhaps even more 'concrete.'

I could ask, for example,

Why am I writing this book?

and my answer would be

Because I want people to learn MOL.

Then

Why do I want people to learn MOL?

Because it's an effective way of helping people.

And

> *Why do I want people to learn an effective way of helping people?*
>> *Because that will reduce the amount of distress that exists.*

So

> *Why do I want to reduce the amount of distress that exists?*
>> *Because that will make the world a better place.*

Now

> *Why do I want the world to be a better place?*
>> *Because I do* (said with a shrug).

To continue the example ...

> *How am I writing this book?*
>> *Well, I'm setting aside time each night to proofread what I've done and then add to it.*

And

> *How am I managing to set aside time each night?*

> Well, I make sure that, whatever else I've got to do, I leave some time for the book.

So

> How do I manage to leave some time for the book?
>> Well, I work out how much time I have and then divide it up amongst the jobs I've got.

Then

> How do I work out how much time I have?
>> Well, I look at the clock and see what time it is.

And

> How do I look at the clock?
>> Well, I turn my head in that direction and make sure I can see it.

So

> How do I turn my head in that direction?
>> Hmmm, 'how' questions get

quite tricky after a while!

You might also notice that if you start with the answer to the last 'why' question and ask "How?" or start with the last 'how' question and ask "Why?" you'll move in the opposite direction.

> *How can I make the world a better place?*
>> *Well, I could help to reduce the amount of distress that exists.*

And

> *Why do I turn my head in that direction?*
>> *Because I want to look at the clock and see what time it is.*

The fact that our inside worlds are organized in a hierarchy of ever increasingly complex experiences is important when dealing with conflicts. Conflicts occur across at least three of these hierarchical levels. The first level is the symptoms the person is aware of. Irritability, anxiety, low mood, and so on, are all likely manifestations of the lowest level of the conflict. The middle level is where the two opposing Bs reside. Goals of autonomy and acceptance, for example, would be at this level. The highest level is where the conflict is actually being created. Perhaps "living the life I want to live" is the experience at this level. It is this highest level that must change for the conflict to be untangled.

> Did you also pick up that there tends to be a range of options for answering 'how' questions? I could probably answer the question "How can I make the world a better place?" in a number of ways. For 'why' questions, however, there tends to be fewer options. The question "Why do I turn my head in that direction?" seems to have a fairly specific answer. 'Why' questions seem to have fewer answers than 'how' questions.

Thoughts to Hold

- ☐ 'How' and 'why' questions can provide a sense of the hierarchical way in which our desires, goals, wants, and yearnings are organized.

- ☐ Conflicts involve at least three levels of the hierarchy.

Your Turn (if you want one)

Try out the 'how' and 'why' activity on something a bit more interesting in your life than reading this book (unless, of course, reading this book is the most interesting thing in your life at the moment). Maybe start with "Why do you get your children to keep their rooms clean?" and follow those answers for a while. Then turn to "How do you get your children to keep their rooms clean?" Or perhaps "Why do you get out of bed at the time you do in the morning?" and "How do you get out of bed at the time you do in the morning?"

Chapter Five

An Untangling Tool

How do conflicts resolve?

So far, so good. Life is control. Problems of living are problems of control. The control problem behind significant chronic psychological distress is conflict. When people are distressed they need to remove conflicts in order to experience satisfaction and contentment again. The removal of conflicts, therefore, is a priority.

Unfortunately, many perfectly good

> With conflicts, it's not that one side is dysfunctional or irrational and the other is functional and rational. Both sides are perfectly valid and legitimate from particular points of view. It's because both sides are entirely legitimate and functional in certain ways that logical methods of problem solving won't work. If there was a logical way of experiencing these opposing states simultaneously, you wouldn't be in conflict!

problem solving strategies are perfectly useless when it comes to conflict. The trickiness of a conflict is that there *is* no way to logically think yourself out of it. No detailed cost/benefit analysis will do. Brainstorming won't cut it either.

For as long as the conflict is in place, no existing solutions will move it. What is needed is a novel solution. A new perspective. An original slant on things. A way of looking at the problem afresh. It's a cruel irony that when we did this sort of learning best we were too young to remember it. Babies spend almost their entire time learning new ways of experiencing the world.

In the first few years of life the amount of learning that goes on is staggering. We acquire the capacity to control an astounding range of experiences. Clearly, babies don't spend their time weighing the pros and cons before they take their first wobbly steps. Nor do they plan their specific sequence of gurgles based on the opinions they think others will form of them when their utterances are heard.

The PCT explanation for the learning that occurs at this basic stage of human development (and the learning that occurs for much less complex beings) is a process of reorganization. When the ability to control is less than satisfactory, and the gap between what is experienced and what is expected can't be closed for important physiological and biochemical states (like body temperature or blood oxygen levels), a random tweaking of the necessary control systems begins and continues until one of the consequences of a tweak has the effect of reducing the gap. The control systems will remain in this newly reorganized state and will only be tweaked further if, at some stage down the track, the gap once again begins to widen or a new gap appears.

> Sometimes a tweak can restore control satisfactorily but conditions might change after some time. Perhaps the person gets married or moves to another town or has some other significant change in circumstances. With changes such as these it might be the case that the tweak that was effective in one situation will need some re-tweaking in a different situation. That's not something that needs to be planned for ahead of time. The reorganizing system will know if further adjustments are necessary.

Since this tweaking involves a reorganizing of control systems the result is the acquisition or development of capacities and capabilities that didn't previously exist. Because the changes are made randomly, there is no guarantee that the best solution will be hit upon first. Have you ever been mulling over the details of a problem and been aware that some of the possible solutions that pop into your head seem over the top, extreme, or even bizarre? In fact, there may be some further deterioration in control abilities for a period of time. Have you ever followed your tennis coach's advice and changed the grip on your forehand only to find that, for a while, you couldn't hit the ball as well as you did before? As the process continues, however, there is a guarantee that a satisfying solution will eventually be found. The particular time frame that is needed, however, can't be specified in advance. Different people learn and reorganize at different rates and in different time periods.

When people are in conflict, therefore, they need help to re-

> It's not usual in this business to offer guarantees but such is the nature of the reorganizing system. The reorganizing system doesn't know good or bad or right or wrong. It doesn't think in terms of social niceties or what other people might think. Its only concern is to reduce error. For as long as this intrinsic error exists, reorganization will keep doing its thing. That's what it's designed to do – guaranteed!

organize. Reorganizing, however, only ever occurs on the inside where people live. No one can see another person's control systems reorganizing, even though you might experience some of the consequences.

In the final analysis (and we've only barely started the book!) people only ever change themselves. Only individuals in conflict know when they are no longer in conflict so only the individual can recognize the right solution when it happens along. Helping means doing what we can from the outside to promote reorganization. So, what can we do?

Thoughts to Hold

- Strategies we have learned in order to solve problems won't help with conflicts.

- Reorganization is a simple form of learning that makes random changes to control systems until control is restored.

An Untangling Tool

Your Turn (if you want one)

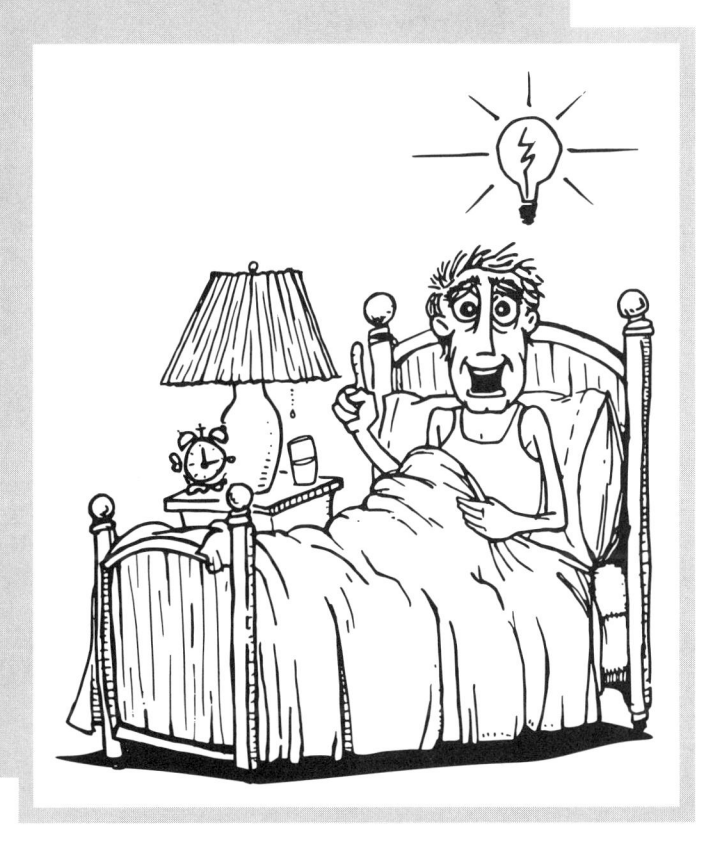

Have you ever had the experience of being unable to solve a tricky problem, going to bed, then waking up in the morning and knowing what the solution is? Can you think of a time when you were trying to recall something like the name of a movie or an actor? Sometimes you can look up the answer, or go through the alphabet, or use some other strategy. At other times, however, nothing works. Has it happened at these times that later on, while you're doing something else, the answer just pops into your head? Some people call this an "Aha!" moment. That experience of a solution occurring to you suddenly, that you immediately recognize as being right, is like the experience of reorganization.

Chapter Six

Finding the Right Place for the Tool

How can reorganization be redirected?

From the outside, we can't affect the occurrence of reorganization but we can affect where it's going on. The basic idea is that reorganization accompanies awareness. Wherever you're focusing your attention is the place reorganization is occurring.

Remember that conflict, according to PCT, occurs across at least three levels of the hierarchy. When people are in conflict, typically what grabs their attention are the symptoms they're experiencing such as the irritability or the frustration or the despair or the anxiety (the first level). Or they might find their attention constantly drawn to one of the unachievable goals (the middle level). They might be aware for example that they "just want to be accepted by others." Unfortunately, while attention is devoted to these lower two levels this is where reorganization will be aimed. This is unfortunate because reorganizing these lower levels will have no lasting effect on the conflict. The focus of attention needs to be turned to the highest level of the conflict so that reorganization can alter the control system creating the conflict.

> Reorganizing the lower levels of the conflict won't affect the existence of the conflict because of the way the hierarchy of control works. What is controlled at one level is determined by the signal coming from the level above. Trying to resolve the conflict by changing the lower levels is a bit like the tail wagging the dog. The conflict will be resolved when the highest level sends different signals down below.

Where is this important control system? Who knows? The only clue we have is that it's higher than the level of the goals. When people you help say things like "I just want to …" or "I wish I could just stop …" then you know they're not there yet because these sound a lot like frustrated goals.

To be as helpful as we can be, our only task

from the sidelines is to constantly direct people's attention to the levels above where they currently are. We don't need to worry about what level they're at or which one they should go to. The bottom line is: if they're in conflict their awareness needs to go up.

Fortunately, nature has helped us out. Whenever people focus on a particular topic they often experience periodic breaks in their focus. These are often just fleeting little blips but their brevity belies how significant they can be.

When people are talking, they will often interrupt their own flow of words in some way. They might pause or smile or shake their head or slow down their speech (or quicken it) or get louder (or softer) or make a kind of judgment about what they're saying –

> The point about disruptions may be important to dwell on. PCT didn't invent or create these disruptions. Disruptions occur whether you know PCT or not. PCT, however, provides one way of understanding them. Based on this understanding a technique has been developed to harness them in order to help resolve conflict. The technique is MOL.

"That sounds really silly." These little disruptions to the word stream are interpreted (from a PCT perspective) as indicating that, just for a second or two, the person's awareness caught something else. Often, but not always, that something else is at a higher level.

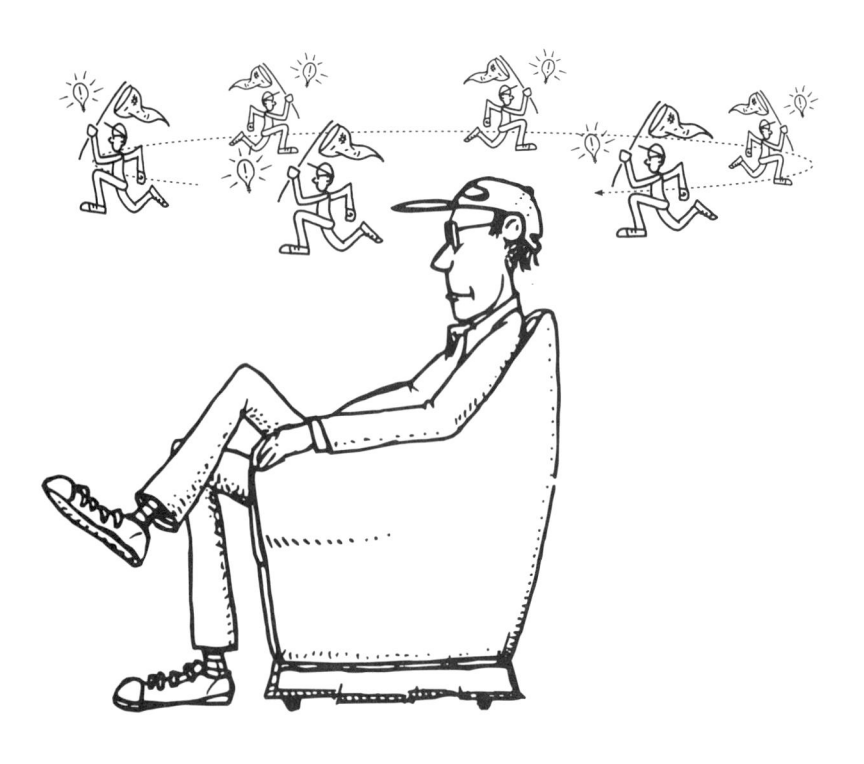

Helping people go up a level, therefore, is more a case of helping them *stay up* once they have had a peek up there themselves. When they indicate to you where that 'up' is — by the little disruption in their word flow — you should help them out by keeping their awareness up there. Essentially, you want to find out what the thought is up there and then get them to hold that thought. Once you know you're working with awareness you can appreciate that your only job is to help people get it up and keep it up.

This can be done by just casually asking things like

- *What's making you smile?*
- *What's going over in your mind as you're slowing your speech down?*

Making the questions present tense will mean that you're helping them catch the higher level while it's still there. If you wait until they reach the end of what they were saying, the place they got to in the disruption will be a faded memory or even forgotten. Helping clients hold onto a thought when one is indicated to you by a disruption is the essence of MOL. Let's look at it some more.

Thoughts to Hold

- [ ] Reorganization goes along with awareness.

- [ ] Brief and subtle shifts in awareness can often be observed as disruptions to a person's flow of speech.

Your Turn (if you want one)

Take some time to go disruption spotting. Turn on the television and watch the news or a chat show or maybe a sporting event. What you need is to be able to observe a period of time where a person is talking on a topic. Interviews are great for this. Watching a politician explaining a new policy or athletes describing their last performance is ideal. During interviews, can you identify times when the awareness of the person being interviewed might have shifted? Maybe they looked away or paused briefly. As you watch, you could practice asking the kinds of questions you might ask in an MOL session if you saw a similar thing happen.

- [ ] What made you pause just then?
- [ ] What came into your mind when you looked away just now?

Chapter Seven

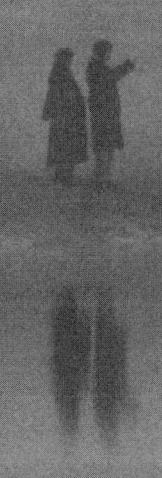

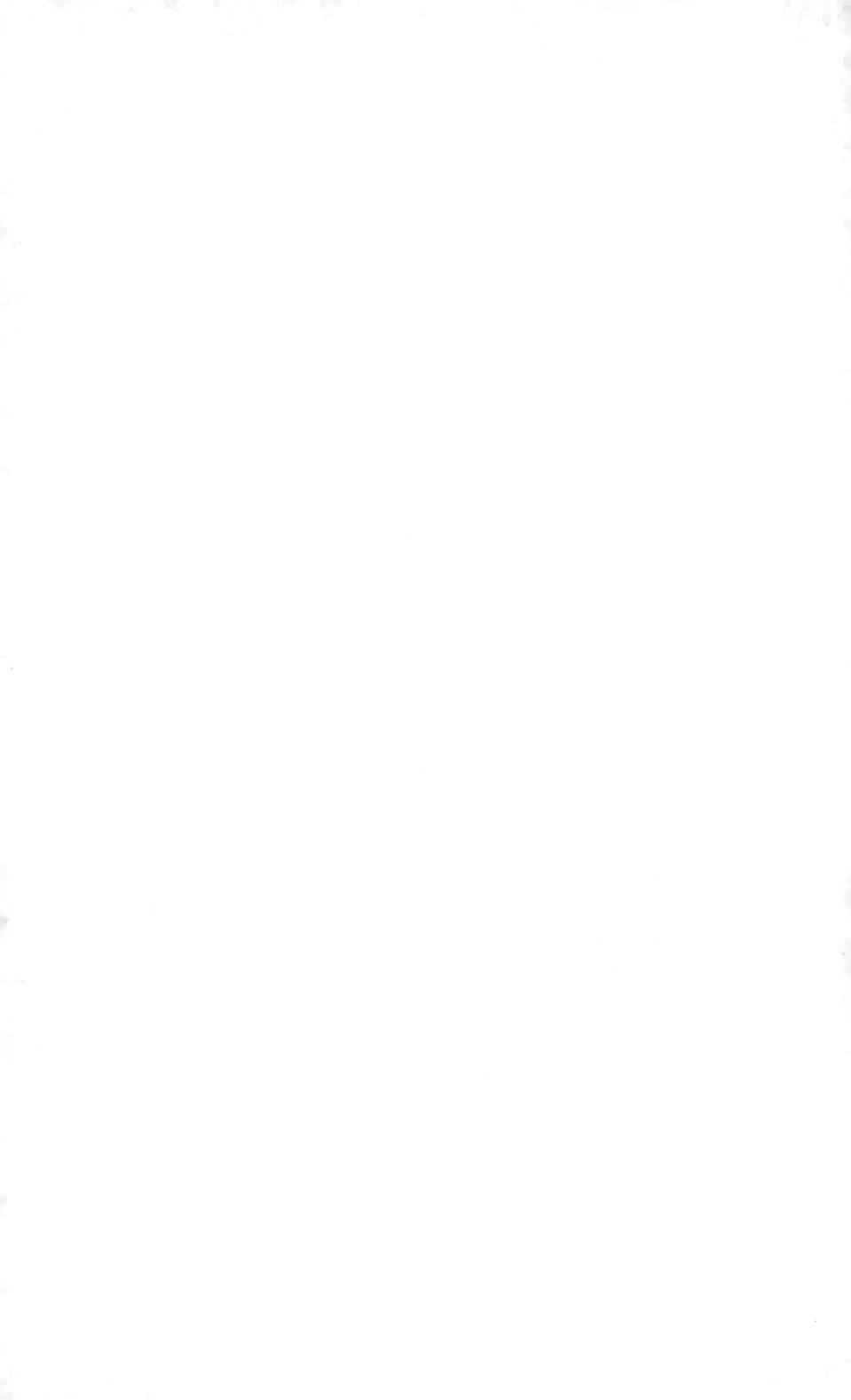

Helping MOL Style

What do people need when they need help?

So that's it. When a person's mind has a conflict, the only thing that will unconflict it is a reorganization at the place where the conflict is being generated. Reorganization will go to work at this place when awareness aims it in that direction. The rule is that the place that gets reorganized is the place that's in awareness.

The neat thing about awareness is that it's always somewhere. So reorganization is constantly tinkering with your being in one place or another. You really are a work in progress. If there's a problem that persists it doesn't mean that reorganization is not going on. It means that reorganization is going on in the wrong place.

When people's problems persist they need help.

> Sometimes you're aware you're aware and at other times you're just aware. Have you ever had the experience of driving somewhere and then realizing your mind had been somewhere else during the driving? Perhaps you were re-playing the successful meeting you just had or imagining your evening tonight in a secluded corner of the restaurant with someone special. So your awareness can be on the job you're involved in at the moment, or on another job while you putter away automatically at the current task ... or even amusing itself with the experience of being aware.

What they need help with though is the place they're looking at the problem from. They don't need help with solutions. A solution that occurs to you as an onlooker to their life is almost certainly not going to be a solution from their perspective as the one who is living the problem. Have you ever wondered why back seat drivers are so irritating? They don't know the driving that's happening for the driver. They only see the view from their position in the car.

People in conflict don't need back seat drivers. They don't need to be told what to do. They need help with where to look for a solution. The solution's not there yet but their reorganizing abilities will create one that is tailor made, custom built, state of the art, and one of a kind. All we can do is help them get to the right place.

Do we know where the right place is? Not when you're the spectator. You just know where the right place isn't. If the conflict is still there, they're not in the right place yet. Sometimes getting to the right spot can take a while. There might be many dead ends and blind alleys encountered before the road that actually does lead to Rome is found. Awareness darts around quickly though, so even with a lot of searching, reorganizing conflicts need not necessarily be a prolonged undertaking. Once they're in the right place change can happen quickly.

> Sometimes it can be frustrating when people seem to be going over and over the same old material or when a solution that seems so obvious to you is not obvious yet to them. That's where an understanding of the strength of the theory can be beneficial. Even though you don't know what the right solution will be for them or how long it will take them to find it, you can be confident that reorganization will keep reorganizing so you just need to help it out by doing what you can to ensure it's reorganizing somewhere useful. The 'doing what you can' involves using disruptions to shove awareness, and therefore reorganization, up to higher levels.

Actually, reorganizing conflicts just takes as

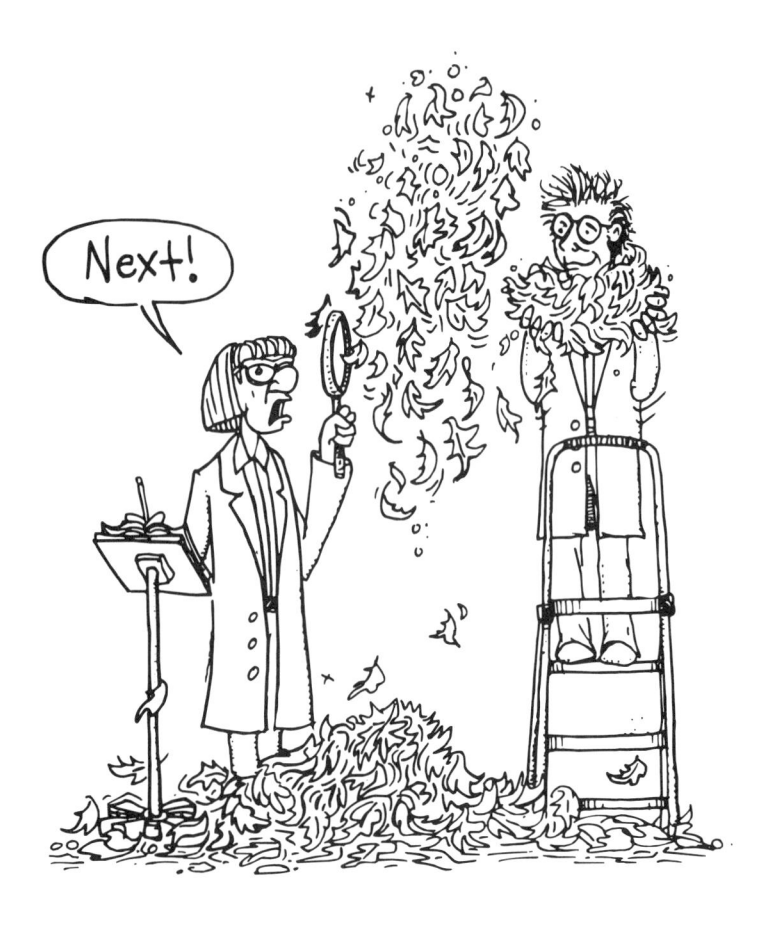

long as it takes. If you're thinking that people should reorganize in five sessions or twelve sessions or before the six o'clock news or in sixteen sessions with a three-month follow-up, you're looking at the wrong thing. Doing MOL means directing people's awareness to higher levels and keeping it there for as long as they need it. It's a bit like throwing armfuls of autumn leaves in the air. You scoop up an armful, give them a heave into the air, and notice how they land. If how they land doesn't work for the person you're helping you throw them up again. You keep throwing them until they land the right way for the other person. That person will know the right way when it appears.

Thoughts to Hold

- Offering help with regard to the resolution of conflict means redirecting awareness to higher levels in the hierarchy.

- The time taken to arrive at a solution will vary among individuals and the solutions will often be surprising.

Your Turn (if you want one)

Some people like to offer advice, suggestions, and supposed solutions to others who are experiencing particular dilemmas. Unfortunately, we seem to find it easier to remember the few times our advice was successful than the many times our advice was rejected. If you're one of these people, count up the number of times that you give advice to people in conflict over the course of a week or so. Of these times, keep a record of what transpires. Do people say "Thank you very much, I'll give that a go" (and do they in fact go on to give it a go)? Or do they offer some reason for why they won't be able to follow your advice or some counterargument for why it won't work? What happens?

Chapter Eight

More About Helping

What's the purpose of asking questions in MOL?

You might have noticed while I've been describing MOL that I've mentioned two things. One is pushing the person's awareness up and the other is keeping it up there. Even though cajoling another person's awareness into more productive places is the key, awareness, like reorganization, only happens on the inside. You can't directly maneuver the awareness of another as though you were rearranging the lounge room furniture.

What you can do is promote the occurrence of disruptions and then make disruptions the focus.

Disruptions are the key to MOL because disruptions are what you can notice from the outside. So your job is to do things to make disruptions more likely and then to ask about them when you spot them. You make disruptions more likely by keeping the conversation happening. By asking about disruptions you'll be turning awareness, and therefore reorganization, to that spot.

In MOL you ask lots of questions. Asking people to explain a little bit more or tell you again about some feature of what they're describing is core business. Assume nothing in MOL. As helpers we tend to assume a lot. If someone says "I just got fired from my job" we assume (sometimes without even knowing that

> The general idea is that you want to know the distressing aspect of whatever the person is describing. Often, we assume that the event being described is just inherently distressing but the distress has to be coming from somewhere. The PCT explanation is that people become distressed when they are unable to control important aspects of their lives. Asking about the distress, therefore, may start to illuminate the important goals, purposes, and values that are currently being thwarted.

we're assuming) that we know how being fired is experienced by the other person. When people say they're depressed or they have panic attacks we assume we know what these mean, too.

Assuming tends to stifle explanation. You don't want to stifle – you want to encourage. So even if you do know how things are for the other person, you pretend you don't. MOL is about being constantly curious. Asking seemingly dumb, simple, obvious questions will get the person talking about the topic. So when you hear "I just got fired from my job" you might reply with things like

> The questions I pose in italics are examples that might help you get started. I don't mean you should ask all of these questions in this order. When I explain something I like to give the general idea so I try and illustrate that general idea with a number of examples.

- *Can you tell me some more about being fired?*
- *Does it bother you that you got fired?*
- *How do you feel about getting fired?*

Or even just

> Fired?

The point of the questions is not for you to find out the answers, it's to get people talking about the topic. You want them talking and you want them looking. As they describe their difficulties to you they'll also be listening to what they say. You might even hear them say things like "No, that doesn't sound right" or "That sounds ridiculous when I say it like that." These are marvelous opportunities to ask them what it is that they're hearing that's not the way they'd like it to sound.

> MOL sessions can feel like hard work for people. Through your questioning they'll be constantly thinking, looking, explaining, describing. By providing them with opportunities to explain in detail the difficulties they're experiencing, without assuming you know what's going on for them, you're more likely to promote conversation that will produce lots of juicy disruptions for you to pluck.

Sometimes getting people to talk is not the problem. Some people seem to be able to talk without the need for regular intakes of oxygen. These people are doing the talking but not the looking. Questions are especially good in this situation. You want to break up what might be a well-rehearsed and often-told story so that they look more closely at the things they're describing. Asking simple, curious questions like

- *Was it blue?*
- *How many times has it happened?*
- *What time of day was it?*

will direct people's attention to aspects they might not have dwelt on before. By considering the things your questions are putting before them, their awareness may start to flit and a disruption will appear.

And that's the point of the questions. You're actually not that interested in the answers to your questions. The questions are for them to explain the story to themselves, not to you. You're interested in the process of their thinking rather than the particular things they're thinking about. So the first task is to create a situation where people will talk about the things that are on their mind. The attitude is constantly tell me more, tell me more, tell me more.

Thoughts to Hold

- In MOL the key to asking questions is to pretend you have no idea what the person is talking about. The general idea is: Assume less, inquire more.

- Although asking questions is the mainstay of MOL, the answers to the questions have little importance. It's people's impressions of what they're saying, not yours, that are important.

Your Turn (if you want one)

Write down the things you think you know when you hear one of these statements:

- [ ] I'm really depressed.
- [ ] My blood is boiling about that.
- [ ] I can't control my anxiety in that situation.
- [ ] Retirement is just around the corner for me.
- [ ] There's a lot of unfinished business from my childhood.

Now identify what makes you so sure of what you think you know.

Find some alone time and take five minutes to discuss a problem with yourself. Maybe driving by yourself in the car would be a good place.

Just think about a problem you're having but instead of thinking about it on the inside, talk about it out loud. What goes through your mind as you hear yourself describing this problem?

Chapter Nine

Ready, Steady, Up

How do you help people delve into the unfamiliar?

Now that you've got them talking, explaining, and describing, you're on the way. As they're filling you in on how all the bits go together you're on the lookout for disruptions. When you spot one you ask about that

- *What stopped you just then?*
- *What made you pause?*
- *What's going through your mind as you glance down?*
- *While you're pausing just now can you talk about what you're thinking?*

Sometimes their pause or sideways glance will be innocuous. "I just remembered I have to go to the bank when I finish here." At other times it will be what you're after. "I was just thinking how much of my life I've wasted." Whenever they mention something that seems to be an evaluation of what they've just been describing that's the thing to hold on to. <u>Thoughts about the thoughts are what you're after.</u>

> They'll hold on to a thought if you help them keep it in their awareness for a time. That can happen just by encouraging them to talk about it.
> - How much of your life have you wasted?
> - What do you think about wasting that much of your life?
> - What do you mean "waste"?
> - How did you decide to waste that much and not any more?

People will have certain thoughts about their problem when they first start talking with you about it. These are probably the thoughts that they've already spoken to their partner, their friends, their goldfish, and the postman about. They are the thoughts they know well. If the conflict is still there, obviously holding these thoughts is not helpful. Your job is to get them to hold other thoughts.

So, whenever a disruption pops up, your job is to get them to try it on for size. Often, if you ask just one question about the disruption they'll answer your question – "Oh, I just thought that I'm the one who's making my problems" – but then they'll go right back to where they were before and continue their story. It's probably good practice to make a point of asking two, three, maybe more, questions about any disruptions that have a hint of a higher level. Questions like

- *What do you mean you're making your problems?*
- *Can you tell me a bit more about that?*
- *How does it sound to you when you hear yourself say it like that?*
- *How long have you been making your own problems?*
- *Do you make all your problems?*
- *How do you feel about making your own problems?*

will help the person stay a little longer at this other place.

As distressing as people's problems can be, the way they currently think about them is familiar. It's also likely to be unhelpful, but there's a certain sense of comfort in what's familiar and the unfamiliar can be daunting. Your job then won't be an easy one. It's not always straightforward to keep nudging people into places they're wary of and yet, to help them reorganize, the places they're avoiding in their minds are probably the places they need to stomp around in for a while.

> Sometimes you might get the idea that there is something the person is avoiding talking about. Asking about that can be useful.
> - Is there something you're wanting to not talk about?
> - Is it difficult to not talk about it?
> - How do you know which are the things to talk about and which are the ones not to talk about?
> - What happens to it when you talk about something else?

This is where focusing on the process of their thinking can be particularly helpful. Sometimes taking a literal approach to the conversation can be a good way of coming up with questions to ask. For example, if people talk about putting things to the back of their mind, or keeping a lid on things, or shutting things away you could ask about two different aspects of these expressions. First, you could ask about the verb part such as the putting or the keeping or the shutting.

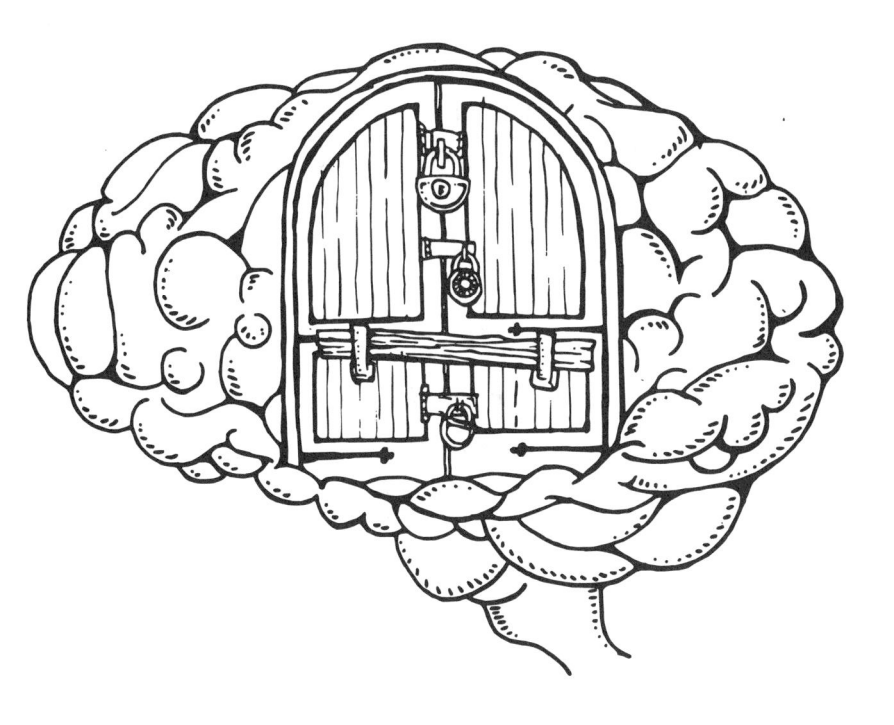

- *Does it take much effort to keep the lid on?*
- *Do you put things in other places or is it always at the back?*
- *How do you put new things in there?*
- *Do you shut the lid gently or*

- with a slam?
- *Do you ever take the lid off?*
- *What's involved in keeping the lid on?*
- *Do you ever bring them back out?*
- *How long would you keep something under the lid for?*
- *Do you ever put the wrong thing back there?*

Or you could focus on the noun parts by asking about the 'thingness' or the location.

- *How do you know which things to put to the back of your mind?*
- *How far back are they?*
- *What is it about the back that makes that a good spot?*
- *Do you ever put them somewhere else?*
- *What sort of a lid is it?*
- *What happens to the things when they're shut away?*
- *Are they still there if you go to look for them again?*

- *Do you have a sense of them even when they're shut away?*
- *What condition does something have to be in for you to shut it away?*

The distinction about verb or noun is not exact and not the important bit of this part of the story. What's important is to keep people talking about the thing that's in their awareness until a shift in their awareness (revealed by a disruption) indicates a new something to ask about.

Thoughts to Hold

- When you hear people make evaluative comments about what they've just been describing these are the thoughts to help them hang on to by asking some questions about the spot their awareness just landed on.

- The process of their thinking is more important than the content. Sometimes asking about the verb or the noun part of their statement can be useful.

Your Turn (if you want one)

Write down five questions you could ask if you heard the following statements (that's five questions per statement!) to help people pause in the place they just arrived at:

- [ ] I don't want to talk about it.
- [ ] That sounds so stupid.
- [ ] There's no point anymore.
- [ ] I always bottle things up.
- [ ] I've always been a failure.

Chapter Ten

Right Here, Right Now

What's the temporal focus of MOL?

When people talk about their difficulties they will almost always talk about events they're regretting or events they're anticipating. They rarely talk about the problem as something they're experiencing *right now*. Trouble is, reorganization can't do anything about past or future goings on. Reorganization only reorganizes what is now, not what was or what is yet to be.

In MOL people

> Time periods other than this very instant will often be important to people because it's generally not this very instant that their distress started. While they might think it's important to revisit the beginning of their distress, if they are still distressed by a past event the distress is happening now. It's the now distress you're interested in helping them transform, not the remembered distress from a previous time.

can talk about whatever comes into their mind. We've already established that what they talk about is not so important. Whenever the conversation has a focus somewhere other than this very instant, however, your helping should involve highlighting the now of their living. This involves nothing more than periodically asking things like

- *What goes through your mind as you revisit these events of your childhood?*
- *How is it for you to picture the future like that just now?*
- *What is your experience of those memories at the moment?*
- *Are there any feelings associated with what you're imagining just now?*
- *Does it bother you to have those images pop into your mind?*
- *What bothers you about that?*

A mechanic would probably find it difficult to

do very much to improve the running of your car if you telephoned in to describe a problem with the car that had occurred last week. When mechanics fix cars they lift the hood and get the engine running. That is, they want to see and hear it running to help them know what to fix. The same idea applies in MOL. With MOL you want reorganization to go where it's needed. To find where that is you need to get the motor running. As much as possible, therefore, people need to talk about how their problem is right now for them as they sit in front of you exploring it.

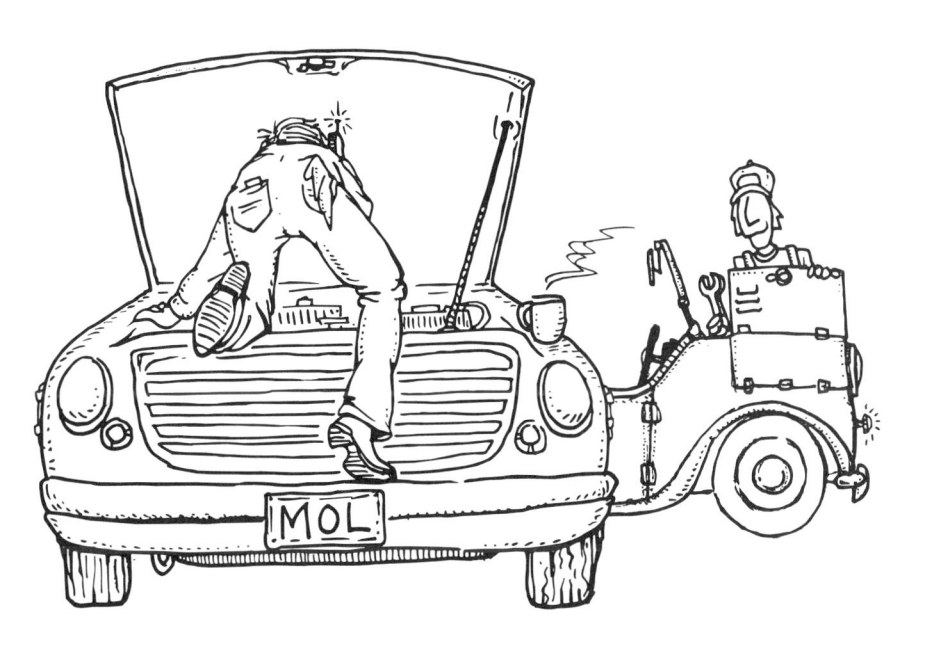

Sometimes, rather than talking about the past or the future, the person might adopt a kind of third person perspective on their problem. When some people discuss their hardships it's almost as though they're talking about someone else. It can seem like they're just watching a movie of their life and reporting on what they see. Adopting a distant, detached perspective may have enabled them to cope with their troubles as they muddle through their life but it's unlikely to be very helpful in reorganizing their conflict.

> Asking about this somewhat removed perspective can sometimes be useful.
> - How would you describe the place in your mind you're recalling things from just now?
> - How do your problems seem to you when you look at them from this place?
> - Do you consider things from this perspective very often?
> - What other things do you look at from the place you're at just now?
> - How do you get yourself to that place?

It can be yucky to talk about painful conflicts. People often spend a good deal of time working out ways to avoid talking about them. It may even be people's very clever avoidance strategies that are the reason the conflict persists. If you don't look at it, it won't go away. Finding out at least a little about the conflict the person is in may provide you with the best clues about where to go next. The things that people bounce off or steer away from, for example, could be the very things they need to look at in order to reorganize.

So the MOL helper's job is to spend the time gently and persistently asking about right now.

- *How do you feel as you describe the week you've had?*
- *What occurs to you as you report those events to me?*
- *What do you think when you hear yourself discussing these things?*
- *What do you make of the experience you've just described?*
- *How do those mishaps sound to you?*

Keeping people talking about things they'd rather not talk about and having them focus on the present when they'd rather be in another time zone are essential aspects of MOL. Sticking to these tasks can be just as awkward and unfamiliar for the MOL helper as it is unsettling for the person seeking help. Adopting an MOL frame of mind will help.

> It is also important, however, that people's autonomy is respected. MOL is not a license to rampage through the private lives of others. People need to know they can always stop the conversation. After some gentle inquiring, if people find talking about particular areas too difficult I would simply end the session with an invitation to resume again when they feel ready. Sometimes explaining to people the importance of looking at difficult areas can help. Not everyone wants to know the reasoning behind the approach being used, but for some people an explanation will be helpful.

Thoughts to Hold

- Reorganization is a present time activity so questioning should constantly return people to the experience they're currently having as they discuss their distress.

- The things people avoid talking about could be important areas to turn their awareness to.

Your Turn (if you want one)

Think about an area of your life that you would not want to talk to another person about and identify what would stop you talking about it.

Periodically throughout the day stop and notice where, in time, your attention is right now. Perhaps put a note on the fridge and each time you see it, think about where your mind is at the moment. Are you thinking about something that happened yesterday or last week or seventeen years, twenty-five days, and three minutes ago or are you imagining events that will occur at some stage in the future. How much of your day do you spend in this moment (and this one, and this one, and …)?

Chapter Eleven

Even Not Having a Topic is a Topic

What do you do when there seems to be nothing to talk about?

In MOL there is always something to talk about. Sometimes, at the beginning of a session, people might say that they don't have anything to talk about or they don't know where to start or they don't know what to say. Don't you find this curious? Is it not a little odd that people would go to the trouble of making an appointment

> Of course, one possibility is that they've changed their mind about this whole therapy thing. Sometimes offering to suspend the session and start again when they feel ready might be the best option. You could ask something like "Are you unsure if this is what you want to be doing?" as a way of helping to decide what to do next.

to see you, get themselves to the appointment, sit themselves down in front of you, and then not know what to say? Can you imagine someone making an appointment to see a dentist for example and sitting down in front of the dentist and saying "I just don't know what to say"?

There are likely to be many possibilities about what might be happening for people who sit down with you and then tell you they don't know what to say. This is an important point to clarify. When people say "I don't know what to say," what do you know? Well, you know that they've just uttered the words "I don't know what to say." You don't know that they *actually* don't know what to say. You just know that they're

> Even after periods of silence you can ask questions.
> - Can you tell me about the silence just now?
> - What was going through your mind as you sat there quietly?
> - Was anything occurring to you while you were silent just then?
>
> The whole point is that you want them to look at what's going on for them. You're not there to figure it out or fix it up, but rather to help them hold it and look at it so they can reorganize it if they need to.

telling you they don't know what to say.

This is a crucial distinction, but luckily in MOL it's also irrelevant. It doesn't matter if people are being straight with you or giving you an account that really should have started with "once upon a time." With MOL it doesn't matter what they talk about because what they talk about doesn't matter. What matters is moving their awareness up.

I find it refreshing and liberating to know that with MOL I don't have to worry about the 'truth' of what people are telling me. The usefulness of the words they utter is in giving you some material to ask questions about.

So, if someone sits down in front of you and says "I just don't know where to start" you could say (bearing in mind that your purpose here is just to get the person talking) things like

- *Tell me about not knowing where to start.*
- *Do you often have the sense that you don't know where to start?*
- *Do you have a number of starting points in mind but don't know which one to*

- pick?
- What is it you're wanting to start?
- Does it bother you to not know where to start?
- When did you first realize you didn't know where to start?

Sometimes during a conversation a similar thing might occur. It can happen that when you ask a person about a disruption you just spotted they might say "I don't know" or "I've gone blank." The same principle applies here. You can be intrigued that someone with a mind in turmoil now, at this moment, reports experiencing blankness or not knowingness.

- Can you tell me about the blankness?
- How do you feel about being blank?
- Does the blankness have a particular color to it?
- Does it have edges?
- Are there any feelings associated with the blankness?

- *What's your experience of not knowing just now?*
- *Is this the same not knowing as the one a few moments ago?*
- *What is it that you don't know?*

With MOL anything can become the focus of curiosity and exploration. If a person asks you "Do you think I'm going crazy?", rather than offering your considered opinion, you might wonder what prompted this question.

- *What made you ask that question just now?*
- *Are you wondering what I'm thinking about you?*
- *Are you concerned that other people generally think you're crazy or is it just my opinion you're interested in?*
- *When did you first start wondering about craziness?*
- *How is it for you to be sitting there wondering if I'm thinking you're crazy?*

The point at every moment is to help people explore wherever their awareness is right now. The point of the exploration is to give you a clue about where to go next. And the clue will usually come in the form of a disruption.

Thoughts to Hold

- [ ] With an attitude of curiosity there will always be something to talk about.

- [ ] The truth or accuracy of what people tell you is unimportant to the process of looking for disruptions and then directing their awareness up.

Your Turn (if you want one)

When I need help generating questions I've found that it can help to think of what people are describing as a physical thing (this is the same as focusing on the 'thingness' that I mentioned in READY, STEADY, UP). For example, when people say "I've just gone blank," think about the 'blank' as something they're holding in their hands behind their backs. Then you could ask questions like

- ☐ How does it feel?
- ☐ Is it heavy?
- ☐ Does it have a color?
- ☐ How big is it?

and so on. The same idea applies when people tell you about feelings they have.

Try it out yourself. Think of something someone told you that had you not knowing what to ask next. Then imagine that what you were told is a physical thing and generate as many questions as you can about its properties.

Chapter Twelve

In the Absence of Disruptions

How do you proceed when disruptions seem lacking?

From time to time it will be the case that the person you're talking with seems to have very few disruptions at all. For one reason or another it will sometimes be the case that it's difficult to find an indicator of where to go next. Having no obvious clue about where to go next can be disconcerting, but with the basic direction of 'up' in mind it's probably useful to adopt an 'anywhere is better than here' mindset.

As people describe their problems to you, you might occasionally ask something like

> *What's running through the back of your mind as you de-*

scribe this situation to me?
- *What thoughts are you having about these events you've experienced?*
- *What's coming into your mind as you remember these things?*

Sometimes there might be an unusual word or phrase that a person seems to keep using. You might also notice a subtle change in people's complexions – such as a faint reddening of their cheeks, or perhaps their eyes mist over ever so slightly as they're talking, or maybe their eyes narrow just a fraction. Anything that catches your atten-

These slight changes can also be thought of as disruptions. The distinction here is that sometimes the word flow is not interrupted when they occur. People sometimes don't miss a beat with the stream of words they're producing even though there are subtle indications that something might be stirring in the background of their mind. It's likely to be helpful to ask about these when you notice them.
- What came into your mind when you narrowed your eyes just now?
- You frowned a little just then; did something occur to you as you were talking?
- What's making your eyes mist over as you speak?

tion may be something to ask about.

The only caution with this approach to directing awareness is that it will be conducted according to your time frame rather than theirs. If you are able to spot disruptions and follow them, then you're probably more likely to be following the contours of the other person's experiential landscape as they're shown to you by the person's awareness. Being guided by people's awareness means you'll be drawing attention to the things that they themselves pick out.

If you ask about background thoughts in the absence of disruptions then the place at which you ask is determined by you and not their awareness. This may not particularly matter in the long run. Going up at all is likely to be better than staying where they are, but perhaps following their lead is more efficient than blazing your own trail. In the course of one conversation there may well be both ways of going up occurring.

Now and then it can be the case that, as the MOL helper, you don't know what to say next. If this occurs it might be more useful to think about your own background thoughts rather than use *What's going through your mind right now?* as a kind of default escape clause. It may be that you've momentarily lost sight of your core tasks with MOL. Perhaps you've started to think of a solution for them or you're trying to figure out what would be best for them or you're wondering if they'll ever improve. These puzzles are likely to distract you from the main business of asking them about what's in their awareness, looking for disruptions, and then asking about the disruption. Being able to go up a level or two yourself by thinking about what your role is might help to get you going again when you feel bogged down.

> While it may not be ideal for you to do the deciding of when the awareness shift occurs, it's not likely to be too much of a problem as long as you're prepared to give up your hunch if it doesn't prove useful. Pursuing a line of questioning because you 'know' there is something there to drag out even though all current evidence indicates otherwise is not likely to be helpful. If your lead goes nowhere it's probably more productive to say something like "I'm sorry, I got us a bit off track there. Where were we?" and then resume the conversation from before while remaining alert to possible new avenues of exploration.

Sticking stubbornly to the task of directing

people's awareness up is possibly the best safeguard against periods of uncertainty. Whether the way up is via their own disruption or your suggestion it's the up that's the key. The destination is more important than the journey.

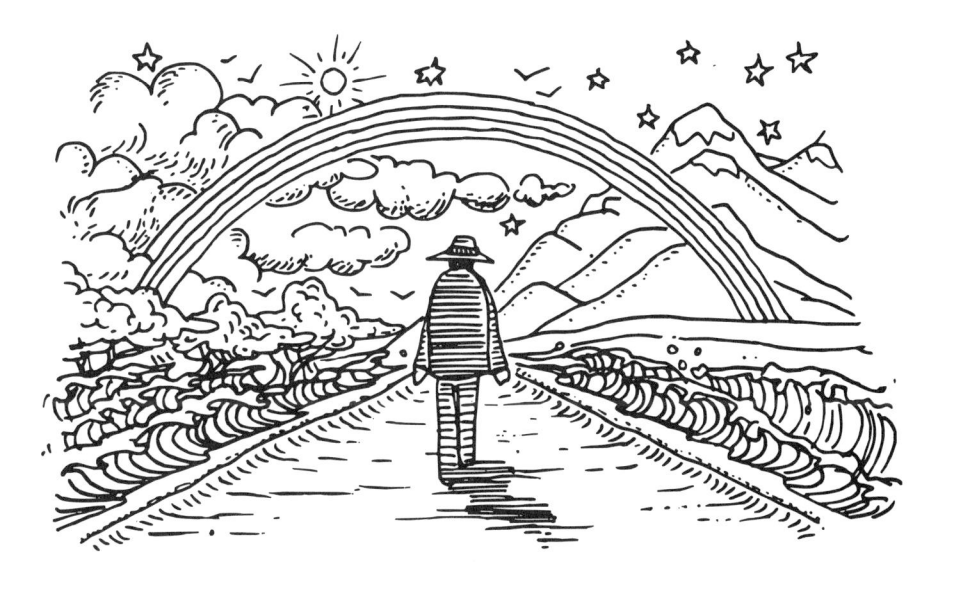

Thoughts to Hold

- When disruptions seem limited it's still possible to ask about background thoughts while being clear that you're hunting for higher levels according to your time frame and not theirs.

- Whenever you feel stumped it might be that you've lost sight of the essential purpose of helping them go up.

Your Turn (if you want one)

Over the coming week, while you're conversing with people, make a mental note of the number of changes you detect in their voice or expressions or postures. They might speed their voice up or slow it down, increase or decrease the volume, start to pause and stammer in a particular place, fall silent momentarily, shift from foot to foot, tighten their grip on the chair, look away, smile suddenly, shake their heads, widen or narrow their eyes, lean in towards you, or put their hand to their mouth. There are undoubtedly other things they will do. What you're looking for is any change in their manner or demeanor as they're talking. Once you get used to spotting these changes it will be easier to figure out what to say at the time.

Chapter Thirteen

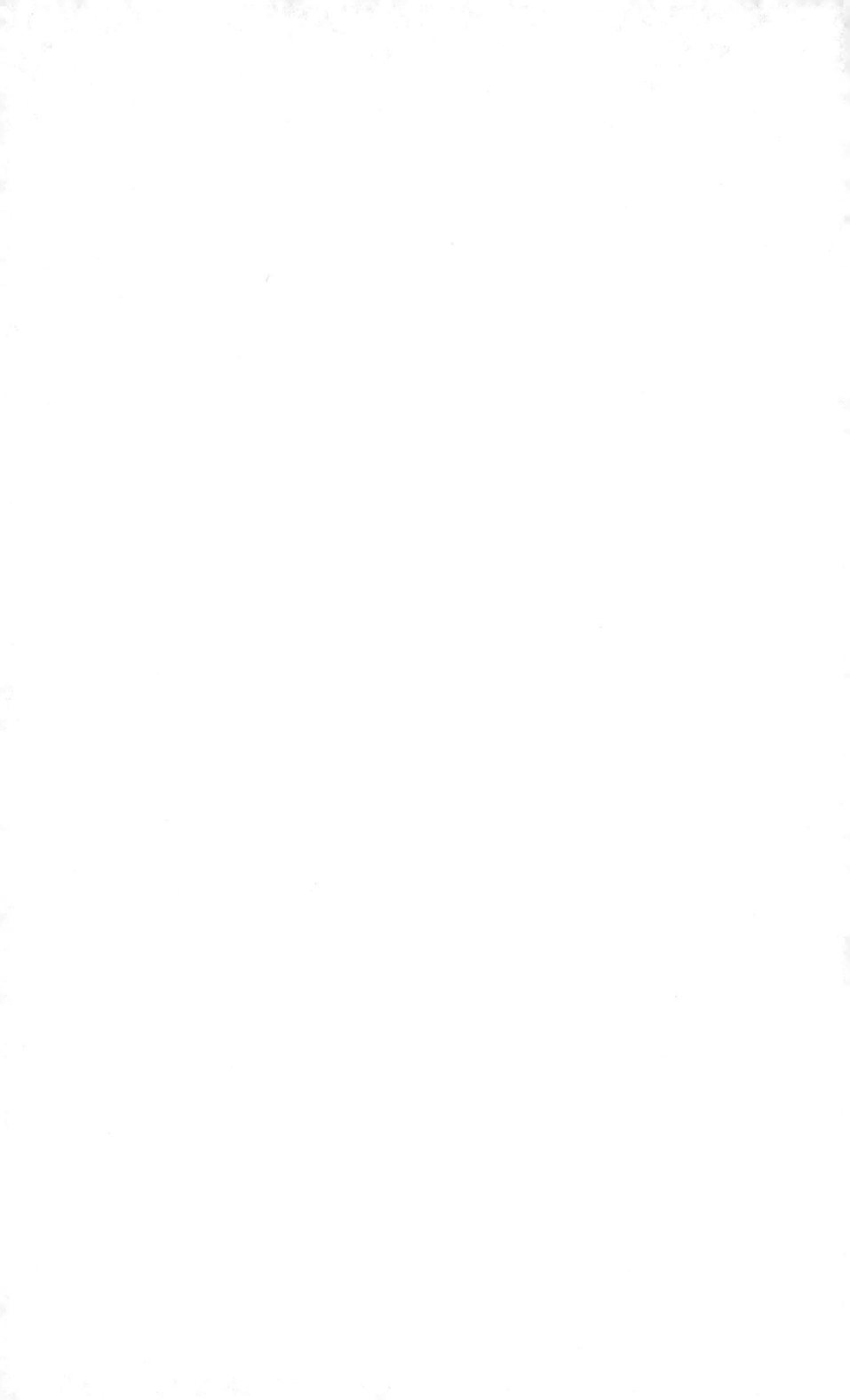

A Special Kind of Helping

What are the goals an MOL therapist should adopt?

MOL helping requires a particular attitude. Being an MOL helper means being clear about the job you have before you. It means setting specific goals and checking at the end of the helping session the extent to which you experienced your goals. As a result of the checking you might modify the goals slightly or focus on different aspects of them.

Helping a la MOL means setting yourself the task of doggedly directing a person's attention to higher places for as long as you're engaged in conversation. This might sound simple but it's not easy. People's stories are often long and involved. If you think it's important to get all the nitty gritty and every itty-bitty detail you will find yourself swamped

> Sometimes my goal for a session will be very specific, such as ASK THREE QUESTIONS FOR EACH DISRUPTION I SPOT and I'll count the questions on my fingers as I ask them. Then I evaluate the session and use the information to inform the goals for the next session I have.
> - Were three questions enough?
> - Did I do it for every disruption?
> - Was it needed for every disruption?
> - What else would have improved the session?

in complexity and despair.

There are two general goals to doing MOL. The first goal is to get people to talk about whatever is in their awareness at the moment. The second goal is to ask about disruptions (or possible higher level thoughts if the disruptions aren't forthcoming). That's it. Once you've done goal two, go back to goal one because now there'll be a new something in awareness that will need exploring. These goals represent the best chance we have of helping someone else reorganize a conflict — at least in a PCT world.

Before every session then it's useful to remind yourself of your job.

> *My job is to ask them about whatever is in awareness*

and notice disruptions.

At the end of the session have a think about how well you did. You might rate, on a scale from one to ten, how curiously you explored their current awareness. You could also rate the frequency with which you picked up on disruptions and the length of time you kept them at the higher level once it snuck into view, or the number of questions you asked in your attempt to get them to hold that thought.

To be an MOL helper I can tell you the goals to adopt but I can't tell you what to do. That would be like telling

> The importance of the therapeutic relationship has long been touted, but it's been much harder to pin down the specifics of this relationship that make the difference. In MOL the defining feature of the relationship is that it's a place where the distressed person feels able to talk freely. It is this aspect that makes the therapeutic relationship different from relationships with friends or loved ones or club members. Mostly, people censor what they say when they talk to others. They couch things in particular terms or avoid certain subjects or leave out uncomfortable details or embellish mundane accomplishments. All these things will impair the ability of awareness to move freely and dwell in trouble spots. When a person can talk without inhibitions or filters, awareness has the opportunity to move where it's needed.

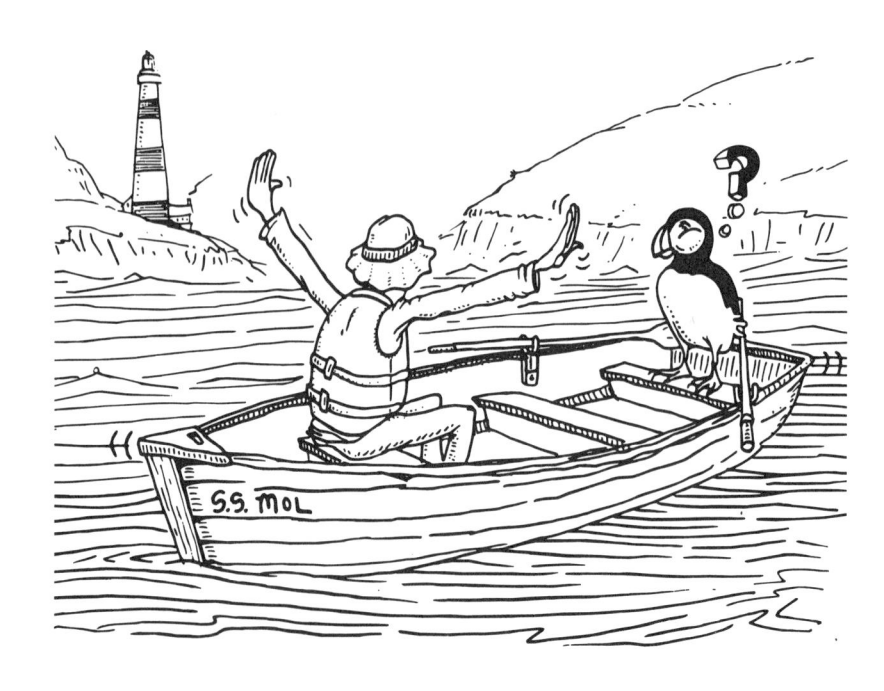

the puffin how many times to flap its wings to get back to its burrow safe and sound.

Goal one is getting people to talk, so do whatever you need to do to let people know you're someone they can let it all hang out with. For MOL to be effective people need to go wherever their awareness takes them. If they're worried about what they're saying to you or how they might appear or what you want them to say, then their awareness will be shackled. Even if they don't tell you what they're looking at, they need to feel OK about looking at it and describing what they see. They need to feel OK about staying with you as you keep them on a difficult topic.

Goal two is to ask about disruptions, so do whatever you need to do to pick up on disruptions and ask a series of questions about them. You need to do this in a way that doesn't shut down the conversation. You need to be able to take people to this new place their awareness has illuminated and have them talk just as freely as they did before.

No doubt we will all go about realizing these goals differently. My MOL sessions will look different from yours. Regardless of the superficial differences, however, we will be doing the same thing in terms of the goals we are pursuing. And it's the goals that make MOL MOL.

> One of the neat things about MOL is that you don't even need to know what the subject matter is in order to ask questions about it. If people have something uncomfortable to talk about they could tell you it's called 'green apples' or 'falling snow' or some other term and you could go along asking questions about green apples with the idea being that you're still looking for disruptions and asking about them in order to move awareness up.

Thoughts to Hold

- [ ] MOL has two basic goals: encourage the person to talk and pick up on disruptions.

- [ ] Sticking to these goals will ensure that MOL therapists are doing the same MOL, even though their specific practices might look different.

Your Turn (if you want one)

The next time you work with someone who is psychologically distressed set the two MOL goals for yourself and evaluate how well you did once you've finished the session.

- What went well?
- What would you do differently?
- Was one goal easier than the other?
- Do you need to make more specific variations of the goal?

Use this information to identify the areas in your MOL practice you might need to focus on next time.

Chapter Fourteen

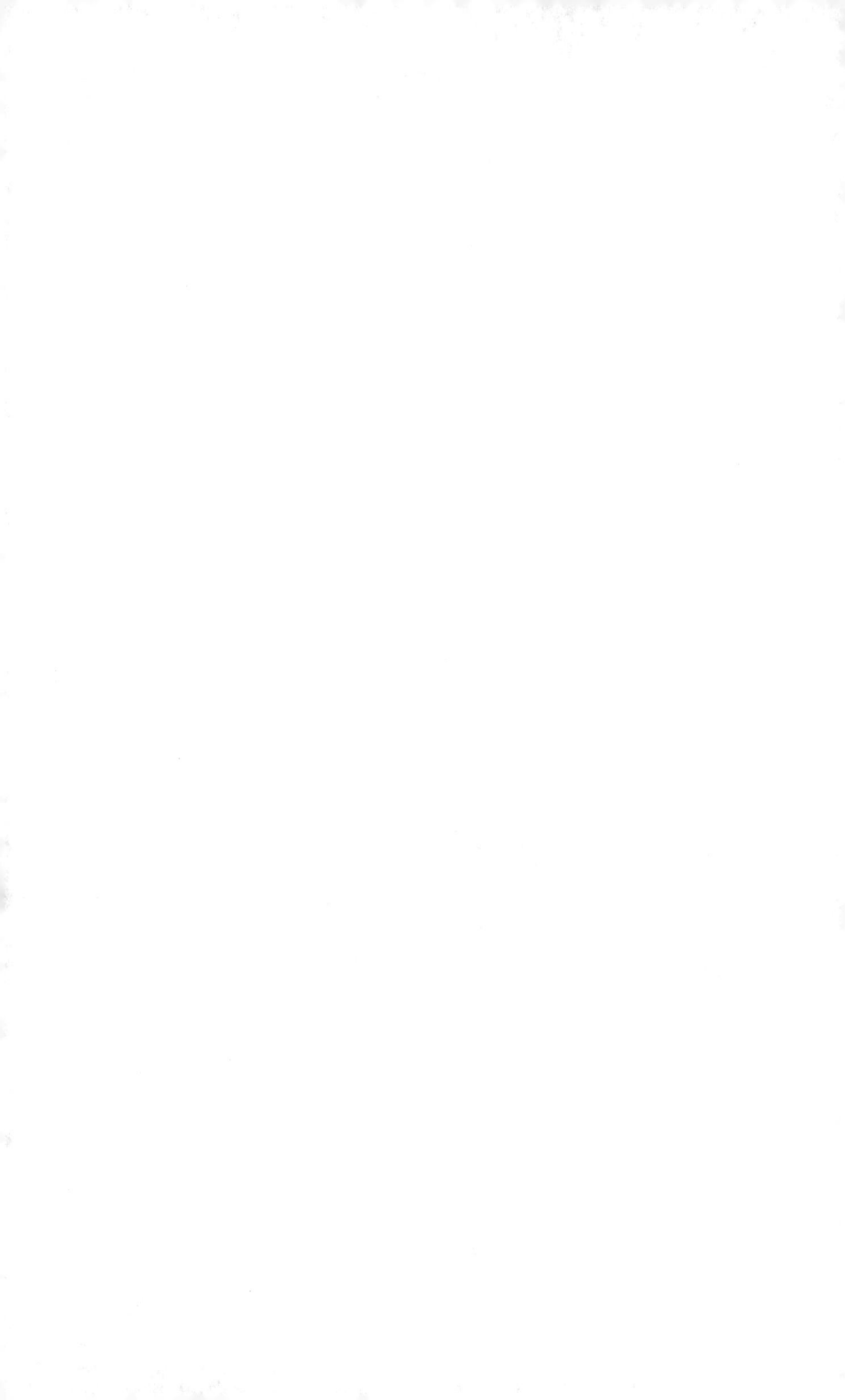

Over to You

Where to from here?

Well there you have it. Life is control — a process of keeping the worlds we sense in the 'just right' states we have specified. Sometimes two 'just rights' will be in opposition with each other. This state of conflict is behind all significant, enduring psychological distress. A process of reorganization will resolve this conflict when awareness is directed to the level where the conflict is being generated. Helping someone who is experiencing psychological distress, therefore, involves directing their awareness up to higher levels. It's as much and as little as that.

I've reached that place in the story where I don't think there's any more I can offer you just now. I hope that by this stage of the book you might

> It can be challenging for therapists when the way people want to live is at odds with the way you think they should live. Unfortunately one person cannot specify the right path for another. We really do have to find our own way through the woods. It has to be our own way because they're our own woods.

have an itch to adopt an MOL attitude, set some MOL goals for yourself, and start hunting for disruptions. I'd like to say there's an easy way to learn MOL but I haven't found it yet.

I still find MOL a slippery little sucker to keep a hold of. That's actually one of the aspects of it I particularly like. You need to be on your toes, stay alert, keep checking on what you're doing. I don't think that's too much to ask when you're playing around in the backyard of someone else's life.

MOL is a profoundly humane and respectful way of helping other people live the lives they want to live. Fundamentally it's a way of helping people that's consistent with the way they are designed. It doesn't get much more basic than that.

MOL is not magic. It won't turn people into superheroes, nor will it make them impervious to the foibles of the world they inhabit. MOL is just about clearing up conflicts. It's about helping people get unstuck so they can return to the business of satisfactory day to day living. Life after MOL might seem like less of an effort, the point of it all might seem obvious again.

You may well feel some trepidation at embarking on this adventure. For many people getting their heads into an MOL attitude will require that *they* reorganize. They might feel the same discomfort as the people they will be helping. Sometimes people's ideas about psychological distress and its causes and cures change radically when given the once over by PCT. MOL can seem like starting from the very beginning again, which can be unsettling for people who are experienced helpers. For other people, MOL might seem like an old friend you've been waiting for a long time to show up.

> With PCT providing the theoretical framework, MOL redefines what it means to be therapeutically useful. This redefining, however, like a new pair of shoes, might take a while to get comfortable. Perhaps you will learn something about yourself and your beliefs about living as you consider these ideas.

What more can I say? Here's MOL ... I know you're gonna have a great time together.

Thoughts to Hold

- [ ] MOL is a way of treating people that fits with how they're designed.

- [ ] MOL can challenge strongly held beliefs about the nature of psychological distress and the purpose of helping.

Your Turn (if you want one)

What are you waiting for?

Check These Out If You Want to Know More

WEB SITES

www.iaact.com

www.livingcontrolsystems.com

www.mindreadings.com

www.perceptualcontroltheory.org

BOOKS

Carey, Timothy A. (2006). *The Method of Levels: How to do Psychotherapy Without Getting in the Way.* Hayward, CA: Living Control Systems Publishing.

Powers, William T. (2005). *Behavior: The Control of Perception* (2nd ed.). New Canaan, CT: Benchmark Publications.

Powers, Willliam T. (1998). *Making Sense of Behavior.* New Canaan, CT: Benchmark Publications.

Runkel, Philip J. (2005). *People as Living Things: The Psychology of Perceptual Control.* Hayward, CA: Living Control Systems Publishing.

ABOUT THE AUTHOR
Timothy A. Carey

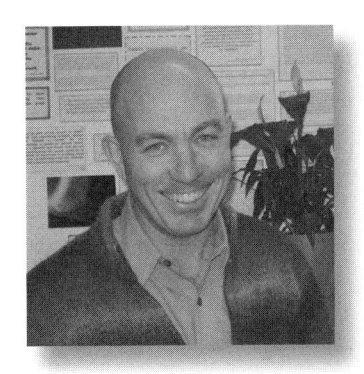

Prior to undertaking studies in psychology Tim worked in schools as a preschool teacher, then a special education teacher and, finally, a behavior management specialist. Whilst completing a PhD in clinical psychology Tim worked in a mental health forensic setting and also correctional centers as well as doing consultancy work in primary and secondary schools regarding approaches to school discipline.

Between 2002 and 2007 he worked in the National Health Service in Scotland as a clinical psychologist in the area of adult primary care. In that time he developed and began evaluating an approach to psychotherapy called the Method of Levels (MOL) which is based on Perceptual Control Theory (PCT). PCT is an intriguing account of how living things function which appeals to Tim's fascination with understanding how things work.

While in Scotland he became interested in the evaluation of psychotherapy generally and the links between research and practice. He also investigated ways of structuring the provision of psychological treatment to maximise client choice and control. Tim's PhD thesis was on countercontrol and he continues to be interested in issues of control in social interactions and in particular its role in the manifestation of antisocial behavior.

After leaving Scotland Tim began working at the University of Canberra where he convenes the postgraduate clinical psychology program and derives a great deal of enjoyment and satisfaction from the teaching, research, and clinical work he does at the university. Working at the university affords him the opportunity to continue learning about PCT and MOL as well as other applications of the theory. It is work that is consuming, enthralling, and invigorating. It could perhaps become all-consuming if it weren't balanced by the magical time of watching with his wife his young son grow and develop in the delightful leafy suburb they share with kangaroos, cockatoos, galahs, magpies, and rosellas.